GROUND FIGHTING TECHNIQUES TO DESTROY YOUR ENEMY

STREET BASED GROUND FIGHTING, BRAZILIAN JIU JITSU, AND MIXED MARTIAL ARTS FIGHTING TECHNIQUES

SAM FURY

Illustrated by
NEIL GERMIO

Copyright SF Nonfiction Books © 2014
Updated 2020

www.SFNonfictionBooks.com

All Rights Reserved
No part of this document may be reproduced without written consent from the author.

WARNINGS AND DISCLAIMERS

The information in this publication is made public for reference only.

Neither the author, publisher, nor anyone else involved in the production of this publication is responsible for how the reader uses the information or the result of his/her actions.

CONTENTS

Introduction	ix
Safety	1
Breakfalls	3
Conserve Your Energy	7
The Ground Position	8
Bringing Your Opponent Down	9

REAR MOUNT

Escaping the Rear Mount	13
Rear Naked Choke	15

FULL MOUNT

Ground and Pound	19
Roll Your Opponent Over	21
Copacabana Choke	23
Arm Triangle Choke	24
The Straight Arm Bar	25
Escaping the Full Mount	28

GUARD POSITION

Guillotine	33
Arm Triangle Choke From the Guard	35
Straight Arm Bar From the Guard	36
Kamura From the Guard	37
Escaping the Guard	38

SIDE MOUNT

Side Mount to Full Mount	43
Kimura From the Side Mount	44
Side Mount Arm Bar	45
Escaping the Side Mount	46
Escaping the Headlock	48

ANKLE LOCKS

Heel Hook	51
Straight Ankle Lock	52
Toe Hold	53
References	55
Author Recommendations	57
About Sam Fury	59

THANKS FOR YOUR PURCHASE

Did you know you can get FREE chapters of any SF Nonfiction Book you want?

https://offers.SFNonfictionBooks.com/Free-Chapters

You will also be among the first to know of FREE review copies, discount offers, bonus content, and more.

Go to:

https://offers.SFNonfictionBooks.com/Free-Chapters

Thanks again for your support.

INTRODUCTION

This book focuses on basic no-gi ground fighting techniques and strategies that are enough to beat inexperienced/beginner ground fighters on the street and in competition.

It's preferable to stay on your feet in a street fight, but many times, you'll end up on the ground, so knowing how to ground fight is an important skill to have.

Some techniques in this book are great for street fighting, but "illegal" in competition. If you plan to use this information for sport fighting, you need to determine what techniques you can and cannot use depending on your discipline and competition rules.

SAFETY

Follow these safety guidelines to get the most out of training while staying uninjured.

- Use proper equipment where applicable (mats, training weapons, protective equipment, etc.).
- Wear appropriate clothing. Don't wear jewelry.
- Train for reality, but only use enough force to get the desired effect.
- Put safety before pride. "Tap out" before you need to.
- Don't train with injuries.
- Get injuries checked out by a professional ASAP to prevent them from getting worse.
- Ensure you're physically ready before you begin training. If you have any doubts, see your physician.
- Warm up, cool down, and stretch.

Tapping Out

Tapping out is something you can do when you submit/give up, like when a lock hurts you. Tap your opponent at least twice, so he feels it. He must disengage immediately. If you cannot reach your opponent, tap the floor. A verbal tap, like "stop," also works.

Chokes

When applied correctly, a choke can cause unconsciousness within 10 seconds.

Disengage the choke as soon as your opponent goes limp or as soon as your training partner taps out. Applying the choke for too long after your opponent is unconscious will cause brain damage, and eventually death.

In most cases, your opponent will regain consciousness within 30 seconds.

BREAKFALLS

Whether you're pushed, tripped, thrown, or you fall, a breakfall will lessen the impact.

The side breakfall is the most common, but it is also important to learn the front and back versions.

The technique for each is different, but there are two major things to remember:

- Do not stick your hand down. This is a natural reaction, but channeling the impact of the fall onto a single point will cause injury.
- Protect your head by angling it away from the ground as you land.

Practice your breakfalls on soft but firm ground such as grass or gym mats. Do it often, so they become instinctive.

Once you are proficient, train doing breakfalls in realistic scenarios, such as when you're being pushed or thrown to the ground.

Side Breakfall

From a standing position, step forward with your right leg and do a single-leg squat as you bring your left leg through. The more you bend the leg, the closer you'll be to the ground before landing.

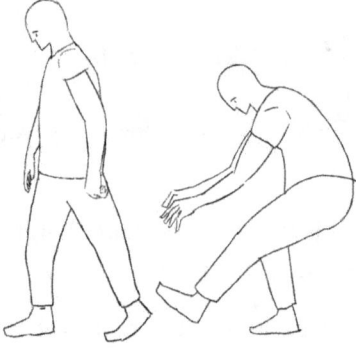

Get as low to the ground as you can, tuck your chin to your chest, and fall onto the left side of your torso/back. You'll also land on the whole of your left arm, which should splay out at about a 45-degree angle from your body, palm facing down. Your legs will probably go in the air.

Breathe out as you hit the ground.

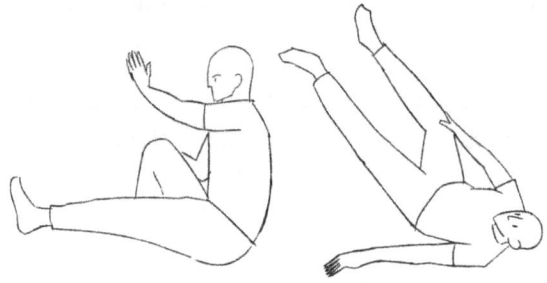

Allow your legs to come back to the ground, finishing in a comfortable position, but not with them splayed too wide or crossed.

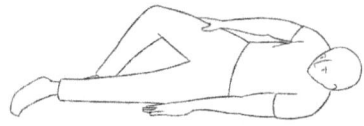

Back Breakfall

Squat down as low as you can and tuck your chin to your chest.

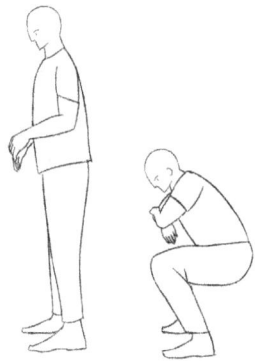

Fall onto your back and arms. Don't roll back too much.

If you stop the roll dead, it will put too much pressure on your body, but you don't want your legs to go too far towards your head for the same reason. To help control this, turn your feet out a little and keep a slight bend in your knees.

Your arms should splay out at about 45 degrees.

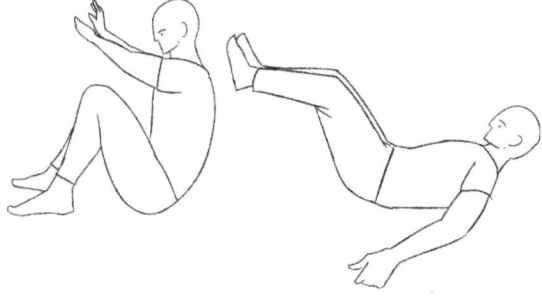

Forward Breakfall

With the front breakfall, you fall directly forward and land on your forearms.

Start on your knees, so you're low to the ground. Put your arms in front of your face in an upside-down V. As you fall towards the ground, tense your core and take the impact on your forearms. Try not to let your belly hit the ground. Turn your face to the side if you have time (not pictured).

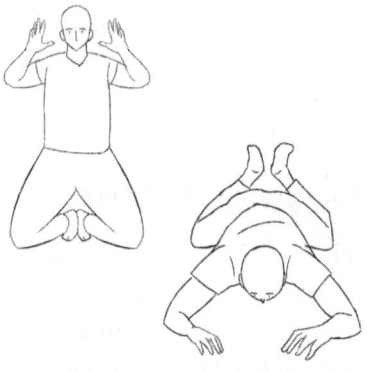

Once you're confident, do it from a standing position. Spread your legs so you can be lower to the ground.

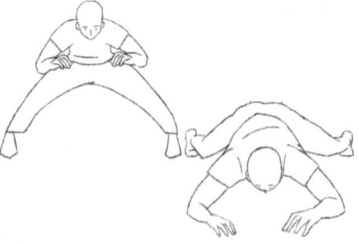

Eventually, you'll be able to do it from a full standing position.

CONSERVE YOUR ENERGY

A ground fight may last a while, and if it drags on, the winner will be the one with the most endurance. To better your chances of winning:

- Take your time and observe your opponent.
- Let him wear out.
- Avoid using brute strength.
- Feel his body and use his movements to your advantage.
- If you find yourself in a position where you're "tied up," don't waste energy struggling. Get your legs free first, then your arms.

THE GROUND POSITION

When your opponent gets you on the ground while he's still standing, adopt the ground position.

As soon as you hit the ground, swing your feet to face your attacker. Use one arm to defend yourself and one leg to kick at your opponent if he comes towards you. Use your other hand and foot to scoot away from him until you have enough distance to get up.

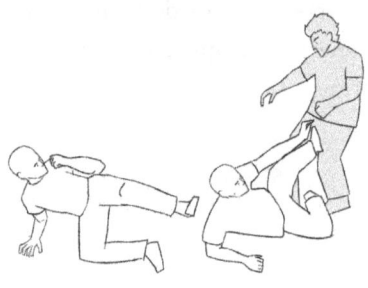

Getting Back on Your Feet

When the timing is right, swing your feet behind you. Use one hand to push yourself up off the ground and the other to protect your face as you stand.

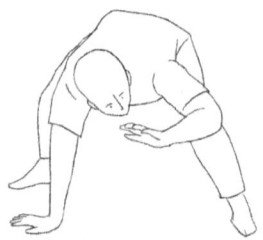

BRINGING YOUR OPPONENT DOWN

When your opponent gets past your kicking feet (or if you want to bring him to the ground), you need to grab his legs. As a kick comes in, or when he gets close enough, grab his leg (preferably both) and hug it/them tight at his knee(s). Lean all your weight at a downward diagonal angle at his thighs to bring him to the ground.

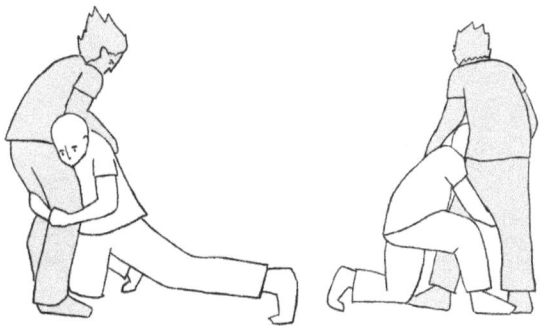

REAR MOUNT

The rear mount (or back mount) is the best position to be in during a ground fight. In this position, your opponent is face down on the ground, and you're either on top of him with your legs hooked under his thighs, or sitting on his back. From here you can strike him until he is out.

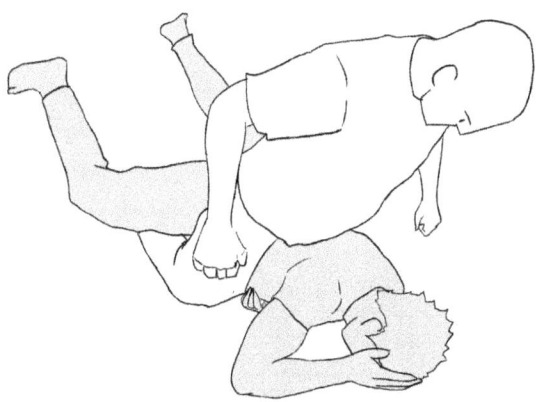

You can also do a back mount when your opponent is sitting up. Wrap both your legs around him and hook your heels on the insides of his legs. Do not cross your ankles. Hold him tightly around his neck.

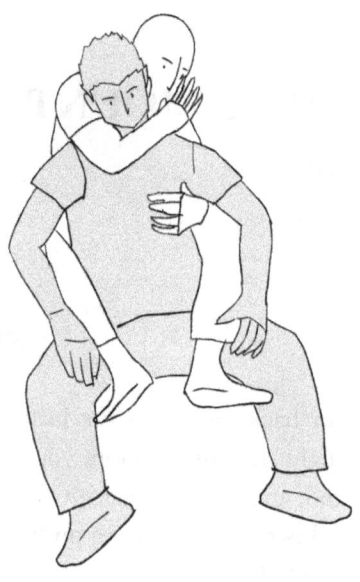

ESCAPING THE REAR MOUNT

When caught in a rear mount, immediately grab your opponent's arm to prevent him from applying (or reapplying) the rear naked choke (see the following chapter).

Position yourself so that your opponent is underneath you—that is, so you're both facing the sky.

The side of his body where his arm is not around your neck is the open side. In this example, it's his left side. Get your foot on the outside of his foot on the open side.

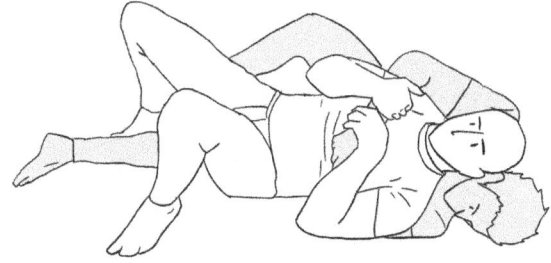

Use your arm to pull his head next to yours on the open side of your head.

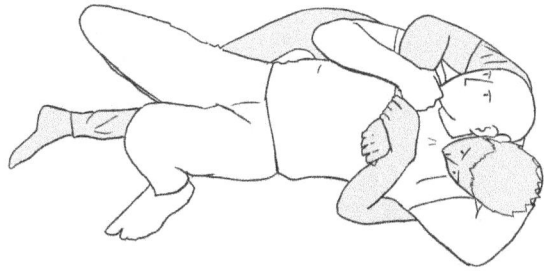

Roll over to your open side to escape the rear mount.

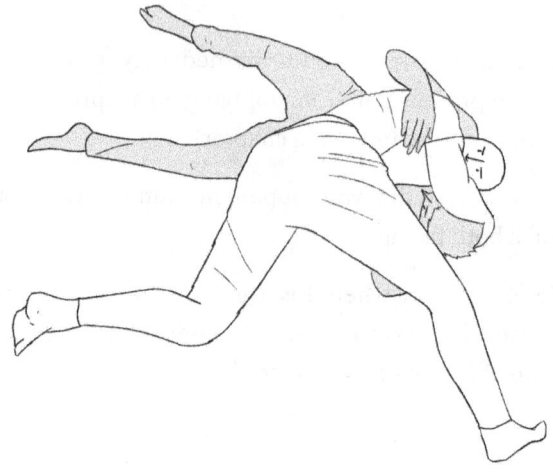

Either stand up or adopt the full or side mount.

Related Chapters:

- Rear Naked Choke

REAR NAKED CHOKE

From the rear mount, apply the rear naked choke (RNC) to take your opponent out.

Place the crook of your elbow over his trachea. If your left arm is around his neck, grab your biceps with your left hand. Put your right hand behind his head and squeeze your elbows together.

If needed, force him to expose his neck by pulling up at his eyes or scraping your forearm under his nose.

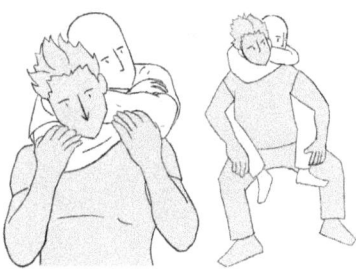

Escaping the RNC

When an RNC is on tight, it's almost impossible to get your head out. You must act fast.

Do what you can to tuck your chin to your shoulder. For example, use your arms to jerk down on your opponent's forearm. This is to free your airway.

In a street fight, attack his eyes, groin, and fingers. In competition, attack his leg. This can also work in a street fight. Grab his foot with both hands, or place your elbow on the inside of his calf and wrench his foot up against it. The hope is that the pain will cause him to let go before you lose consciousness.

If he crosses his ankles, put the underside of your knee over his top foot and apply downward pressure.

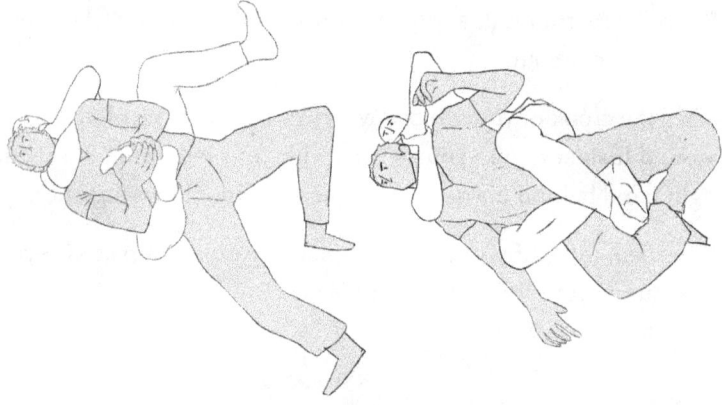

FULL MOUNT

When you can't perform a back mount, do a full mount. Sit on your opponent's torso, so you're facing him. Get your knees as close to his armpits as possible.

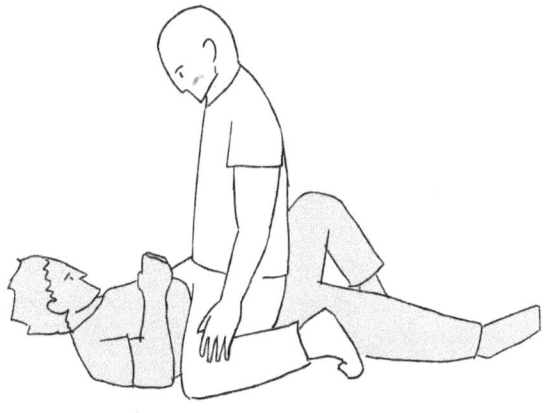

If you need to, limit his movement by:

- Squeezing his midsection with your thighs
- Put your feet underneath his hips
- Holding his head

Use your arms, elbows, and head to stabilize yourself.

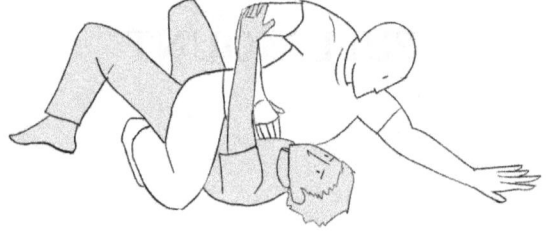

GROUND AND POUND

Once in the full mount, you can continuously strike your opponent until he's out.

Be careful to not lose your balance as you strike. Angle your elbows across his face/head, so that if you miss, you don't smash your elbow into the ground.

When you want to keep your distance, use hooking punches.

If he turns to protect himself, let him, and then adopt the rear mount.

Forming a Fist

A proper fist will allow you to punch without injuring yourself.

Hold your hand out flat, with your fingers together and your thumb up.

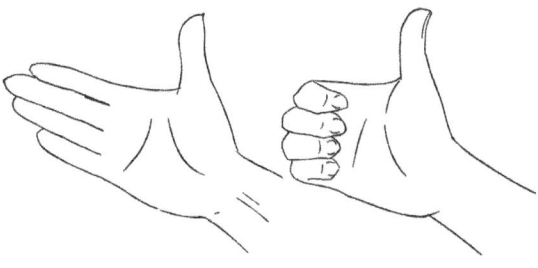

Roll your fingers into your palm and then bring your thumb down over your fingers.

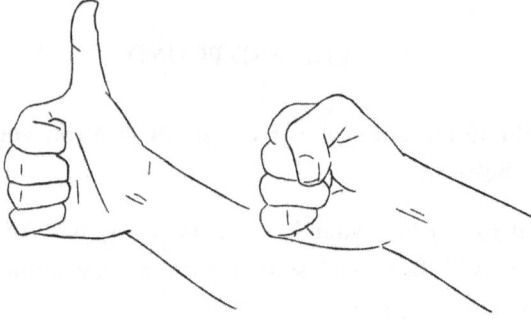

Hold your fist loose until just before it makes contact. You need to have relaxed muscles to produce speed and power. This is true for all strikes.

Alignment of your wrist is important in all punches. Angle your wrist up to align your fist with your forearm. If it connects while it's bent down, you'll get injured.

As long as you hold your fist correctly, you can strike from any angle.

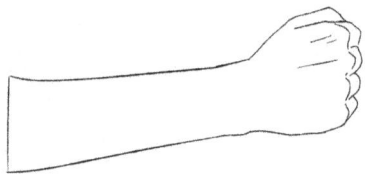

ROLL YOUR OPPONENT OVER

When your strikes aren't getting through, or you don't want to strike, try to roll your opponent over.

Use both of your hands to push one of his arms across his body, and lean down on it.

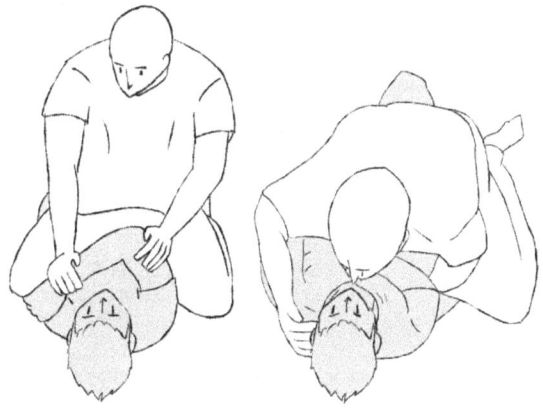

Reach around his head and grab the wrist of the captured hand.

Place your free hand on his elbow to hold him in place.

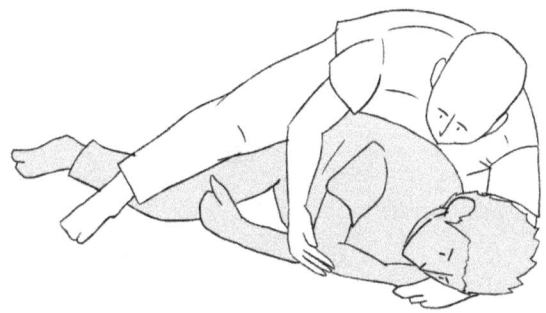

Reposition yourself so you can use your chest to force him over and adopt the rear mount.

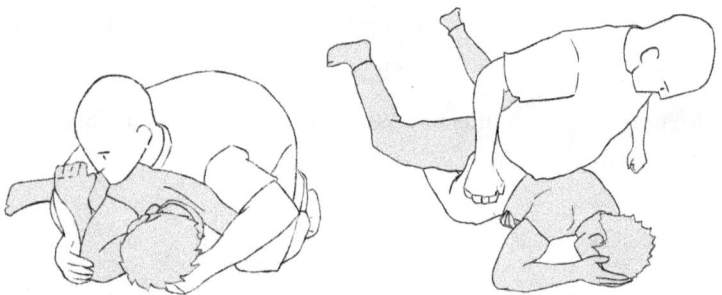

COPACABANA CHOKE

The other option besides striking or rolling an opponent over is to choke him out.

To do the Copacabana choke, lean forward so most of your weight is on him (without losing your balance). Place one hand behind his head. Make a V with your other hand and place it on his trachea. Pull his head up as you drive your body forward. To conserve energy, it is important that you use your body to apply the pressure, rather than your arm.

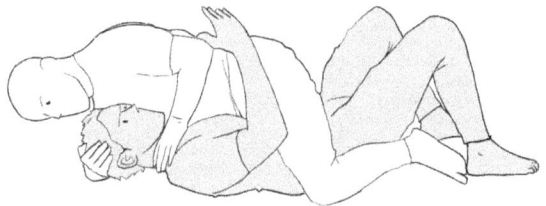

ARM TRIANGLE CHOKE

To apply the arm triangle choke, place one arm behind/under your opponent's neck. Grab your wrist with your other hand and pull him in tight, so the side of your head squeezes his neck against your upper arm.

It works better if his arm is between your head and his neck, as this narrows the gap more.

Alternatively, use your shoulder and opposite fist to squeeze his arteries.

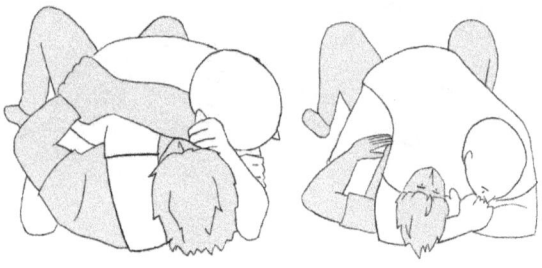

You can apply this move from the side or behind, on the ground or standing, though the RNC is more effective.

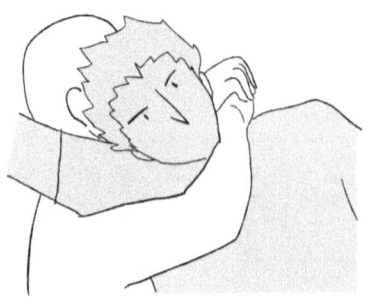

THE STRAIGHT ARM BAR

When you're in a full mount and your opponent tries to push you off, apply the straight arm bar.

If you want to grab his right arm, place your right hand on his chest, in between his arms. This will isolate the arm. Put your left arm around the outside of his right arm and place it on your right hand.

Lean your weight on his chest, then swing your left foot around the top of his head. Sit down as close as you can to his shoulder. Do not fall back yet. Sit up and hug his arm.

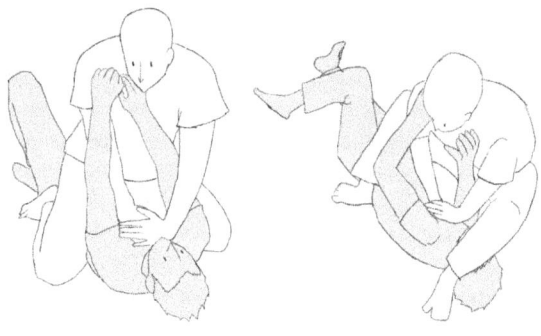

Cross your ankles and squeeze your knees to clasp his arm. As you lie back, shift your hands up to grip his wrist. Raise your hips and pull back on his arm.

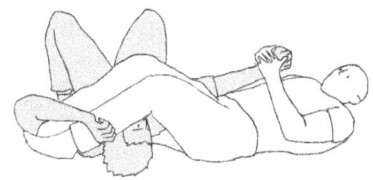

Escaping/Preventing the Straight Arm Bar

To prevent the straight arm bar, do everything you can to put your hands together in a monkey grip. Put your fingers against his knee and push it up, over, and off your head/face.

Use your legs to drive your body back until your head has his leg pinned to the ground. Push on the ground with your feet to lift your hips off the ground.

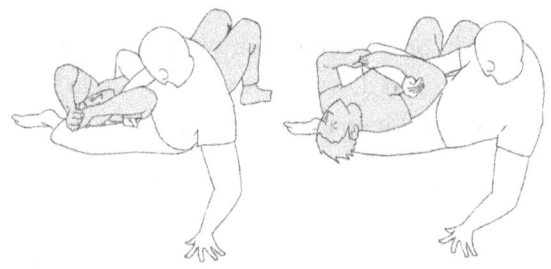

Spin in hard towards your opponent to end up in his guard.

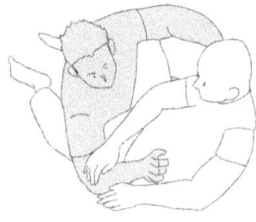

Hitchhiker's Escape

When you are not fast enough to grip your hands together, use the hitchhiker's escape.

As your arm is getting extended, turn your thumb towards whichever one of his hips is closest to your head. Use your other hand to hold his ankle in place.

Roll back over your shoulder, bringing your feet over his foot.

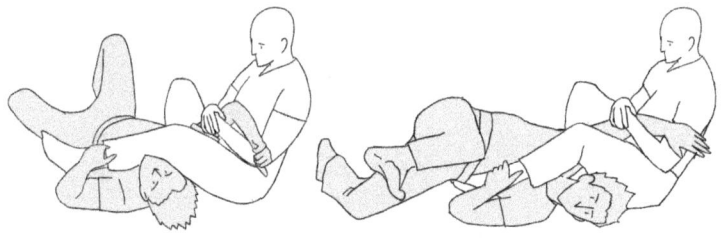

He may or may not roll over with you. Either way, continue to roll over until you're on your knees, and then adopt a mount position (rear, full, or side).

ESCAPING THE FULL MOUNT

In a street fight against an inexperienced fighter, a simple eye gouge and/or groin grab can be enough to get him off you.

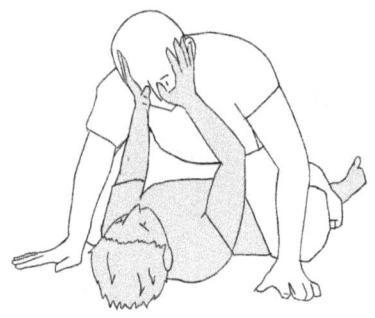

Upa Escape

When the eye gouge and/or groin grab is not an option, try the upa escape.

Hook one of your feet around the outside of his and grab his arm on the same side. This is the trapped side.

Buck your hips to direct him forward and over to the side you trapped. This will flip him over so you're in his guard.

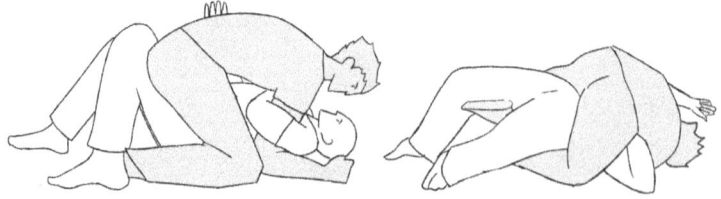

Elbow Escape

When the upa escape is not possible, use the elbow escape to put him in your guard.

Do your best to control his arms as you lower your guard, to prevent him striking you.

Turn on your side, with your leg flat on the ground. Hold his leg in place and bring your knee through the opening.

Once your knee is past his leg, put your weight on the same leg. Turn towards the other side so you can pull your leg out and wrap it around his back.

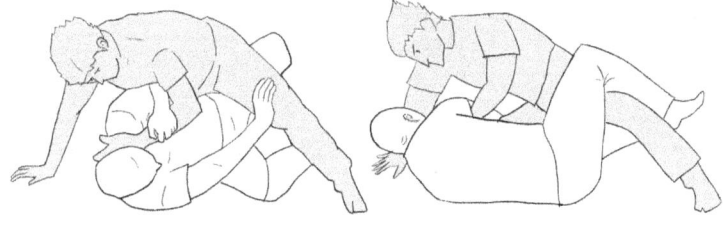

Repeat the movement on the other side to put him in your guard.

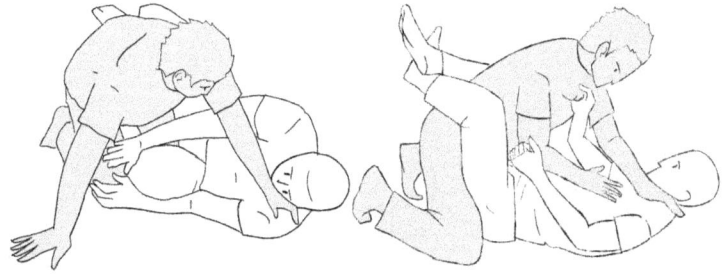

GUARD POSITION

When you end up on the bottom in a ground fight, putting your opponent in the guard position is the best thing to do. Cross your legs around his waist and use your hips to control his distance.

In most cases, you will want to pull him in tight to prevent him from striking you. Pulling him in close also allows you to attack.

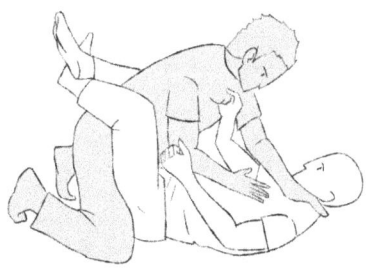

GUILLOTINE

The guillotine is an excellent way to take out your opponent from the guard position.

Wrap your arm around the back of your opponent's neck and under the front of it. His head should be to the side of your torso.

Your palm should face your chest, so the top of your wrist cuts into his throat just below his Adam's apple.

Use your other hand to grasp your first hand.

Push him away with your legs while pulling his neck towards your chin.

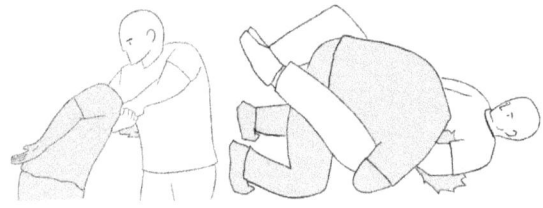

Escaping the Guillotine

To escape the guillotine, act quickly before your opponent crosses his ankles and pulls you in. Attack his groin and eyes.

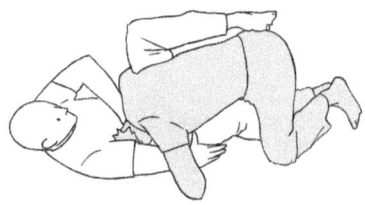

If attacking the eyes and groin doesn't work, place your hands on his thighs to prevent him from rolling on top of you as you escape.

Forward roll over your shoulder on the side that your head is on.

Roll back in towards him to free your head, then adopt the full or side mount.

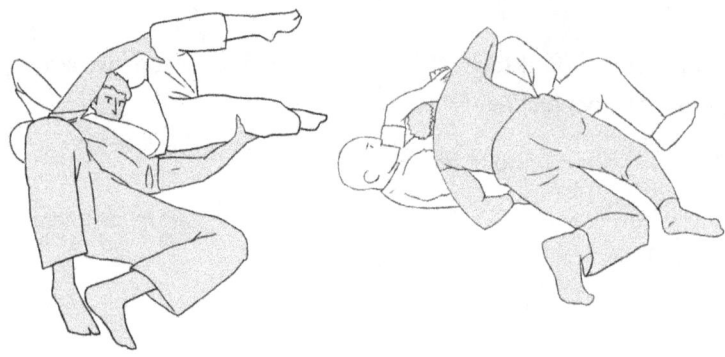

ARM TRIANGLE CHOKE FROM THE GUARD

The technique you use to apply the arm triangle choke from the guard position is almost the same as the one you use to apply it from a mount.

For more leverage, grab the back of your head with your non-choking arm, then grab the bicep of that arm.

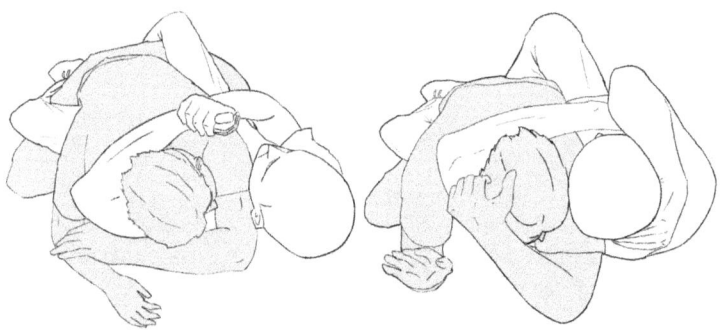

Related Chapters:

- Arm Triangle Choke

STRAIGHT ARM BAR FROM THE GUARD

Adapting the straight arm bar from the guard is a good alternative to a choke. Capture your opponent's arm to prevent or stop him from striking you.

Release your legs and spin so you capture the target arm between your legs. You can use your hand on his leg to help you spin.

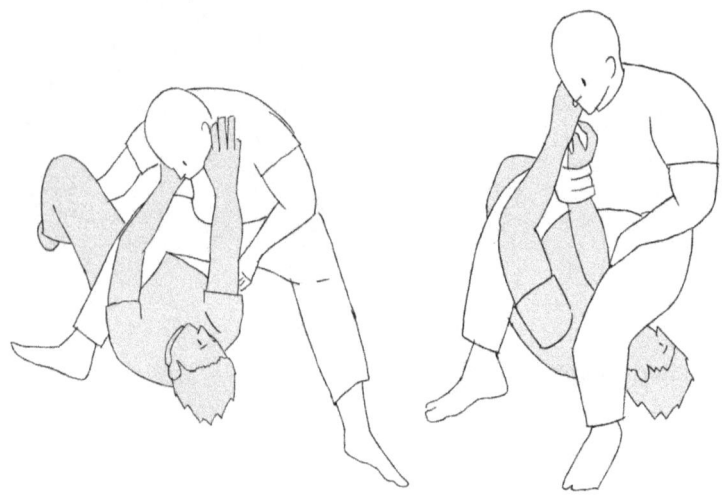

Extend your body to apply the arm bar.

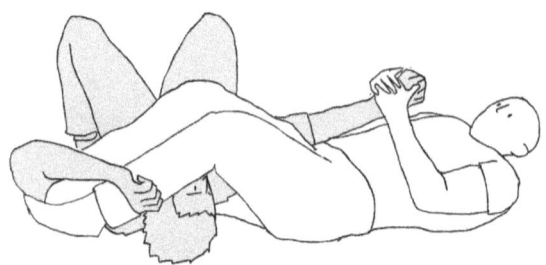

KAMURA FROM THE GUARD

The kamura is a wrist lock.

Grab your opponent's wrist with your closest hand—that is, if you're reaching for his left wrist, use your right hand. Keep your thumb next to your fingers. Place your opposite foot on the ground for balance, then reach over his shoulder and thread your arm under his elbow to grab your own wrist.

Lie back while keeping his elbow tight against your body. Cross your ankles again and torque his wrist towards him as you apply pressure to his arm.

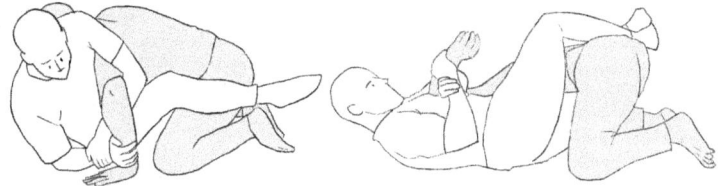

ESCAPING THE GUARD

The first step in escaping your opponent's guard is to strike him. A few solid blows may be all you need.

When he hasn't crossed his legs, move over them into a mount.

An experienced ground fighter will cross his legs and pull you in. In that case, weave your arms inside of his, then sit back. Push on his torso to create distance.

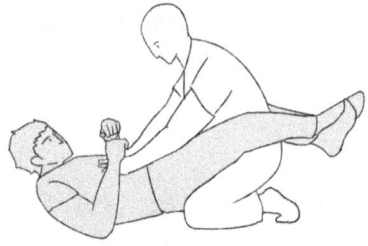

Use stiff arms for support and attack his groin with your knee until he uncrosses his legs. Stand up or pass over his legs into the mount.

Smashing the back of his head on the ground will also work, but is a last resort. It will knock most people out, but can cause brain damage or death.

Stacking Guard Pass

When attacking the groin is not an option, use the stacking guard pass.

Weave your arms inside your opponent's, then sit back. Push on his torso to create distance.

Strike him to "loosen him up" a little so you can under hook his knees with your elbows. Dip one shoulder underneath his knee and cup his shoulder with that hand. Your other hand should hold his thigh.

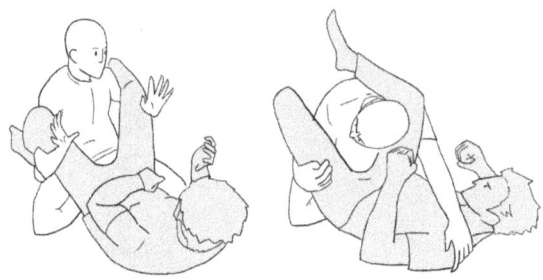

Push forward with your feet to "stack" him. Keep a wide base for balance and turn your head in case he tries to strike you. "Walk" around to the side, keeping your wide base. Lift your head to get around his leg.

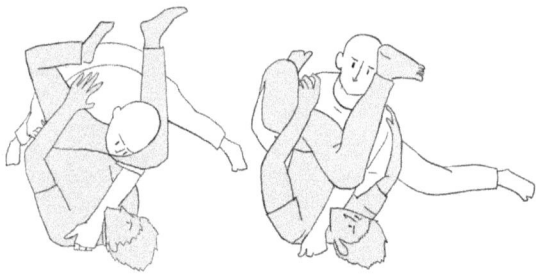

Drop your chest onto him to adopt the side mount.

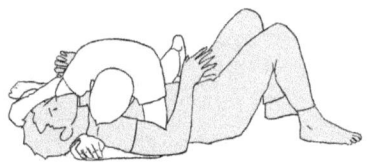

SIDE MOUNT

When you have your opponent in the side mount, he's on his back and you're lying perpendicularly on top of him.

Pass one arm (the one closest to his neck) under his neck and the other arm under his arm, so you can clasp your hand together. Hold him tightly, with your knee up against his head.

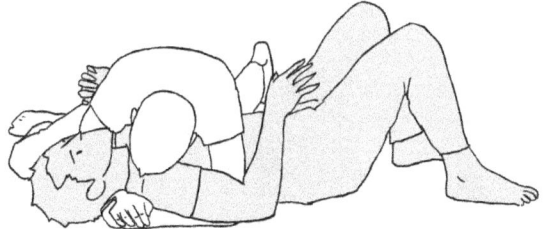

SIDE MOUNT TO FULL MOUNT

In a ground fight, you want to get to a rear mount. To do this from a side mount, you first need to get to a full mount.

Place your knee across your opponent's thighs/lower abdomen. Use your arm to push his legs down if you need to.

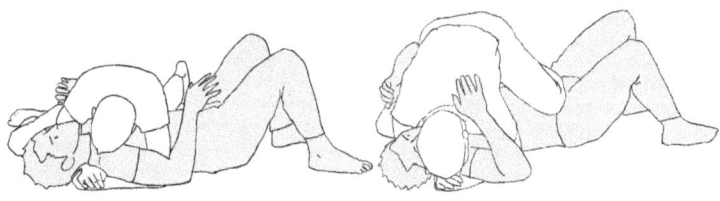

Slide your knees as close to his armpit as you can. Place your foot down to the ground to adopt the full mount.

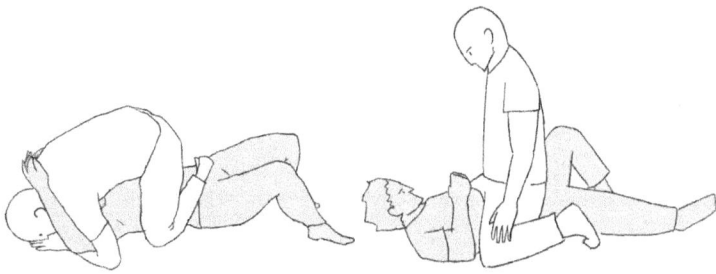

From the full mount, you can roll him over to the rear mount as described in the full mount section.

KIMURA FROM THE SIDE MOUNT

You can apply the kimura arm lock from the side mount.

Assuming your left hand is closest to his legs, place your left hand behind and up against his left hip. This is to keep him from moving his hips.

Move your right arm under his right arm and use your head to pin his lower right arm against his body. Most of your weight should be across his chest.

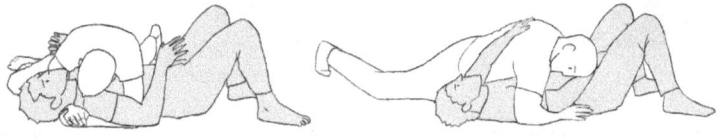

Bring your left hand up to grab his right wrist, then weave your right hand under his elbow to grab your left wrist. Once your hands are in position, put both your elbows flat on the floor.

Shift your weight forward and step over his head with your right foot. Keep his arm held tightly against your body. Use your left hand to torque his arm away from you, "brushing" his hand across the floor.

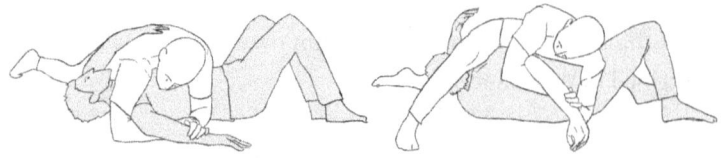

SIDE MOUNT ARM BAR

Another arm submission technique you can do from the side mount is the side mount arm bar.

Put your knee on your opponent's torso or neck to pin him down. Extend your other leg for balance.

Capture his arm by wrapping your arm around it at his elbow. This is the wrap arm/hand.

Place your non-wrap hand on his shoulder. Grab the wrist of your non-wrap arm with your wrap hand. Arch back to apply pressure to his arm.

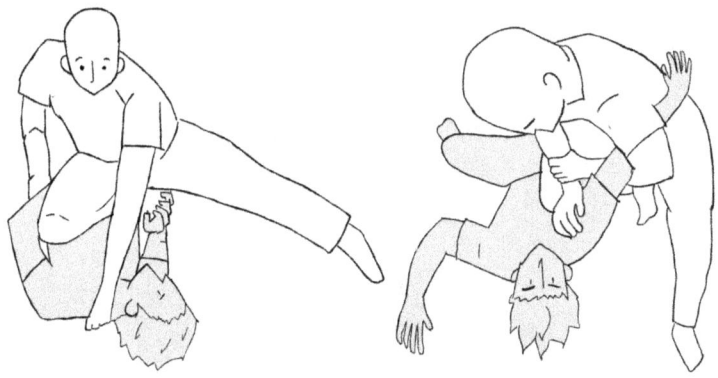

ESCAPING THE SIDE MOUNT

When the side control is loose, use a groin grab and/or eye gouge.

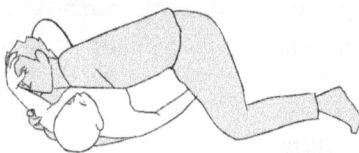

From a tight side control, your aim is to get your arms inside his guard.

Lift your feet off the ground and get your arms ready to swing.

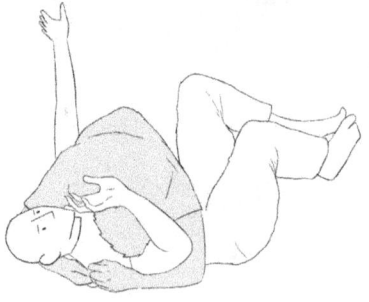

Do the following simultaneously:

- Plant your feet as close to him as you can.
- Swing your arms in a wide circle to "chop" his arms under his armpit and at the crook of his elbow.
- Buck your hip up towards his head.

He may roll over, but it is not likely.

Ground Fighting Techniques To Destroy Your Enemy

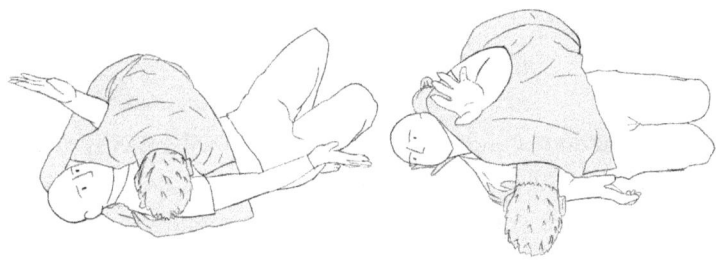

Bring your hands between his through the gaps you created with your "swing and buck" movement. He will settle back, but now your hands will be between his.

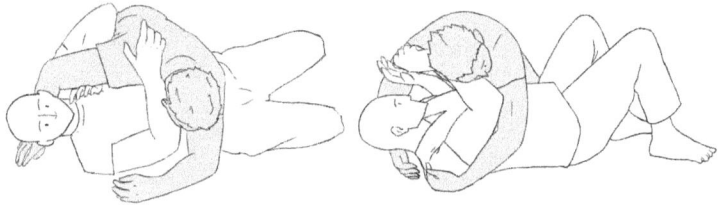

Push him away to create some room. Place your feet on the ground and scoot your hip out so you face him. Drive your knee back in and adopt the guard position.

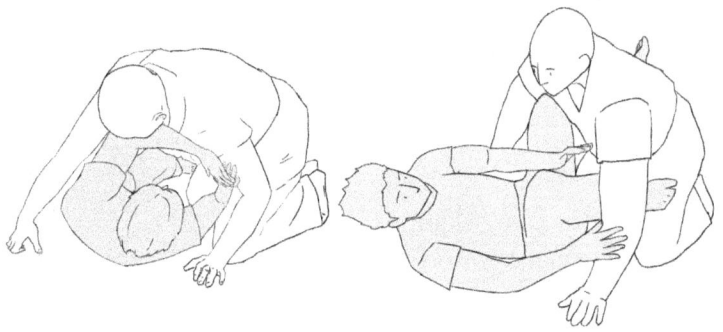

ESCAPING THE HEADLOCK

People that do not know how to ground fight will often apply the common headlock. To escape it, turn on your side to face your opponent. Bring your top arm under his jawbone and hold your wrist with your other hand to form a frame.

Rotate around so you are on your knees at your opponent's back.

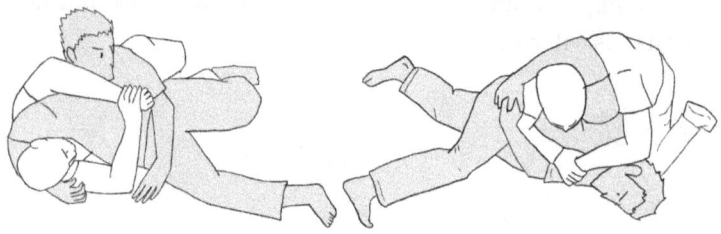

Step over him and apply pressure with your frame until he lets go.

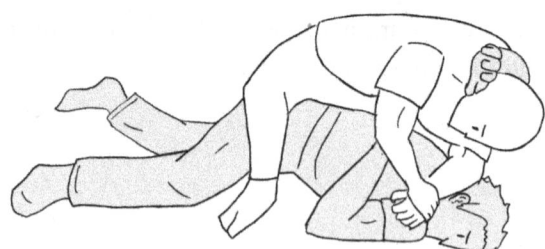

ANKLE LOCKS

Although your goal should not be to apply ankle locks, it's good to know how to do them, in case an opportunity presents itself.

HEEL HOOK

Be careful when using the heel hook in training. Damage is often done before it is felt.

Put both your legs around one of your opponent's, then place his instep against your ribs and hook his heel in your wrist. Immobilize his upper leg and hips with your legs. Turn your upper body to rotate his lower leg. Either his pinkie or his big toe will be on top.

You can also do this when he's on his stomach.

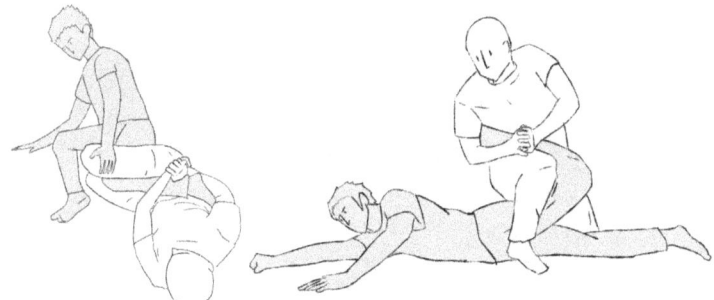

STRAIGHT ANKLE LOCK

To apply the straight ankle lock, place both your legs around one of your opponent's. His foot will be under your armpit. Assuming his foot is under your left armpit, wrap your left arm under his heel. Place your right hand on his shin and grab the wrist of your right hand with your left hand. Arch back to apply pressure.

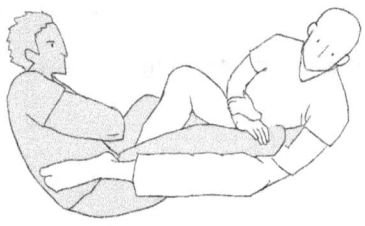

TOE HOLD

The told hold is a versatile ankle lock that you can do from a variety of positions.

Only two variations (of many) are pictured here, but the general application is the same for all.

Grab your opponent's toes with one hand and use your other arm to wrap under his ankle. Use your wrapping hand to grab the forearm of your toe-holding hand. Push his toes towards him to apply pressure.

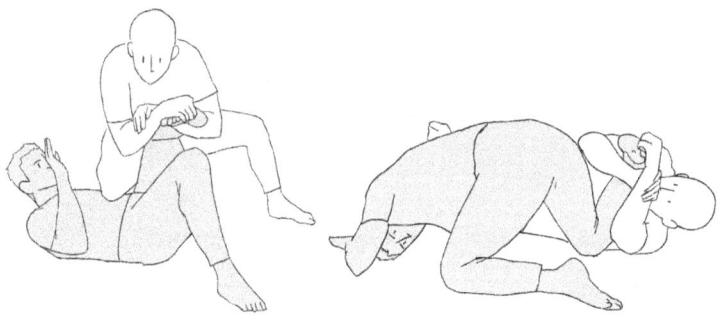

THANKS FOR READING

Dear reader,

Thank you for reading *Ground Fighting Techniques To Destroy Your Enemy*.

If you enjoyed this book, please leave a review where you bought it. It helps more than most people think.

Don't forget your FREE book chapters!

You will also be among the first to know of FREE review copies, discount offers, bonus content, and more.

Go to:

https://offers.SFNonfictionBooks.com/Free-Chapters

Thanks again for your support.

REFERENCES

AppOpus. (2012). *U.S. Army Field Manual FM 3-25.150 (21-150) COMBATIVES: Expanded Edition*. AppOpus.

Cheung, W. (1852). *Dynamic Chi Sao by William Cheung*. Unique Publications.

Filotto, G. (2011). *Systema : The Russian Martial System*. CreateSpace Independent Publishing Platform.

Gracie, C. (2003). *Cesar Gracie Brazilian Jiu-Jitsu & Gracie Jiu-Jitsu Grappling Instructional Series*. Ultimate Imports.

Indio, D. (2012). *Mixed Martial Arts Fighting Techniques: Apply Modern Training Methods Used by MMA Pros!*. Tuttle Publishing.

Jacques, M. (2009). *The Grappler's Handbook Gi and No-Gi Techniques*. Black Belt Books.

Kemerly, T. Snyder, S. (2009) *Taekwondo Grappling Techniques: Hone Your Competitive Edge for Mixed Martial Arts*. Tuttle Publishing.

Lee, B. (2008). *Bruce Lee's Fighting Method*. Black Belt Communications.

Lee, B. (2011). *Tao of Jeet Kune Do: Expanded Edition*. Black Belt Communications.

Lung, Haha. Prowant, C. (2000). *Ninja Shadowhand - The Art Of Invisibility*. Citadel Press.

Mamiko, V. (2012). *Systema No Contact Combat*. Varangian Press.

Plyler, D. Seibert, C. (2009) *The Ultimate Mixed Martial Arts Training Guide: Techniques for Fitness, Self Defense, and Competition.* Krause Publications.

AUTHOR RECOMMENDATIONS

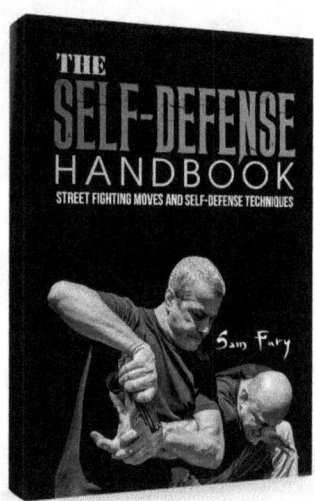

Teach Yourself Self-Defense

This is the only self-defense training manual you need, because these are the best street fighting moves around.

Get it now.

www.SFNonfictionBooks.com/Self-Defense-Handbook

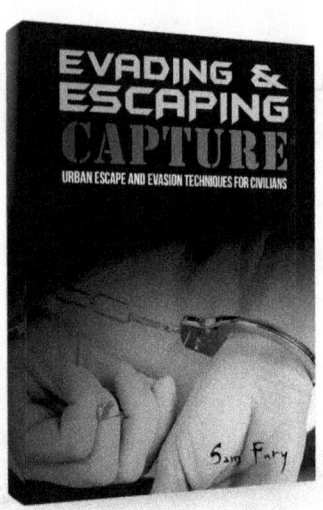

Teach Yourself Escape and Evasion Tactics!

Discover the skills you need to evade and escape capture, because you never know when they will save your life.

Get it now.

www.SFNonfictionBooks.com/Evading-Escaping-Capture

ABOUT SAM FURY

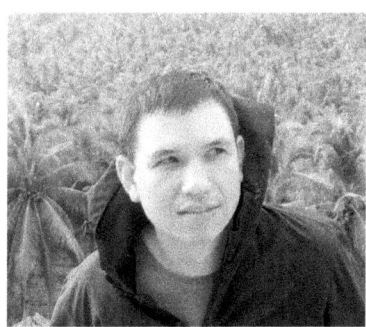

Sam Fury has had a passion for survival, evasion, resistance, and escape (SERE) training since he was a young boy growing up in Australia.

This led him to years of training and career experience in related subjects, including martial arts, military training, survival skills, outdoor sports, and sustainable living.

These days, Sam spends his time refining existing skills, gaining new skills, and sharing what he learns via the Survival Fitness Plan website.

www.SurvivalFitnessPlan.com

- amazon.com/author/samfury
- goodreads.com/SamFury
- facebook.com/AuthorSamFury
- instagram.com/AuthorSamFury
- youtube.com/SurvivalFitnessPlan

www.ingramcontent.com/pod-product-compliance
Lightning Source LLC
Chambersburg PA
CBHW070033040426
42333CB00040B/1671